HMR DIET FOR WEIGHT LOSS

A Structured Meal Plan for Beginners to Achieve Rapid Fat Loss and Long-Term Health

CAROLINE SIMMONS, MD

Copyright Page

Copyright © 2024 by Caroline Simmons, MD.

All rights reserved. No part of this book may be reproduced, stored in a retrieval system, or transmitted in any form or by any means, electronic, mechanical, photocopying, recording, or otherwise, without the prior written permission of the author, except in the case of brief quotations embodied in critical articles and reviews.

The recipes and suggestions provided in this book are for informational purposes only. The author and publisher are not responsible for any adverse effects or consequences resulting from the use of the recipes, dietary practices, or suggestions described herein. Always consult a professional or medical expert if you have any concerns regarding your dietary needs and health conditions.

Table of Contents

Copyright Page 2

Table of Contents 4

INTRODUCTION TO THE HMR DIET 1

How the HMR Diet Works: Basics and Principles

.... 3

HMR Program Options 8

HMR Program Foods 11

What Are the Health Benefits of the HMR Diet?

.... 13

GETTING STARTED WITH THE HMR DIET 16

What Does the HMR Program Cost? 16

Is HMR Program Easy to Follow? 18

Who Should Not Try the HMR Program? 21

Does the HMR Program Work? 22

THE HMR DIET PLAN IN DETAIL 24

Phase 1: Weight Loss Diet................................ 24

Phase 2: Weight Maintenance........................ 26

Further Details on the HMR Diet Plan 28

HMR DIET RECIPES YOU MUST TRY!................ 43

DELIGHTFUL RECIPES FOR BREAKFAST 43

Chicken Mini Frittatas.. 43

Spinach Fritters 45

Tunisian Shakshuka 47

Zucchini, Pea, & Halloumi Fritters 50

Simple Cheese & Veggie Omelet....................... 52

Overnight Cereal in a Jar 54

Pistachio & Grape Yogurt Bowl 56

Cinnamon Roll Porridge With Cranberries...... 57

Cauliflower and Egg Salad 59

Golden Shrimp & Avocado Toast 61

Raspberry and Granola Greek Yogurt 63

Tangy Tuna Sandwich 64

Greek Vegetable Omelet 66

Breakfast Potato Salad 68

Almond Flour Pancakes.......................... 70

DELIGHTFUL RECIPES FOR LUNCH.................73

Mediterranean Chicken Casserole 73

Risotto Peanut Lettuce Wraps 74

Roasted Veggie Mac and Cheese...................... 75

Garlic Shrimp 77

Chicken Salad Wrap 79

Chicken Soup 80

Chicken Souvlaki..................................... 82

Prosciutto and Pesto Sandwich 84

Salmon and Spinach Salad 85

Chicken Wraps....................................... 87

Chili 89

Avocado and Chickpea Salad 91

Avocado Seafood Wraps 92

Orange & Pomegranate Salad 94

Chili Nachos 96

Pasta Frittata 98

Caprese Chicken 100

Prosciutto Salad 102

DELIGHTFUL RECIPES FOR DINNER 105

Shephers Pie Boats 105

Super Spinach Lasagna 107

Whole Grain Medley in Squash 108

Chicken and Broccoli Casserole 109

Chicken Parmesan Meatballs 111

Chicken Rolls 113

Spanish Chicken and Rice 115

Supreme Pizza 118

Chicken, Chickpea, and Pita Salad 120

Turkey Burgers 123

Vegetarian Greek Pasta............................... 125

Zucchini Boats...128

Mudardara and Side Salad............................ 130

Moghrabieh with Chicken.............................. 133

Mediterranean Turkey Casserole 137

DELIGHTFUL RECIPES FOR SNACKS.................141

Fiesta Chicken Burrito Bowl...........................141

Fajita Bowl 142

Chocolate Chunkie Monkie Shake...................144

Cranberry Orange Shake 145

Green Giant Shake 146

Mint Hot Chocolate 147

Pumpkin Pie Smoothie 148

Chili Fries 149

Caramel Apple Shake....................................150

Berry Berry Good Shake...............................151

Berry Banana Parfait 152

Salted Caramel Mocha Shake 154

Strawberry Swirl Shake.................................. 155

Twice Baked Pot Pie Potatoes 156

Vanilla Berry Smoothie Bowl 157

SUCCESS STORIES, TIPS AND REVIEWS.......... 159

Success Stories and Tips from Real People 159

Reviews 162

1

INTRODUCTION TO THE HMR DIET

Health Management Resources, a health and weight loss company, initially developed the HMR Program in 1983 as a diet and lifestyle solution to help people achieve long-term weight loss success.

The HMR program is a dual-phased plan that consists of structured meal plans and behavioral coaching for long-lasting, healthy lifestyle behaviors and habits. Members can participate in the program either at home or in person at a local HMR weight loss clinic.

In March 2023, the company was acquired by Profile Plan, a weight loss solutions and nutrition company established by Sanford Health. Although Profile Plan now owns HMR assets, the HMR program remains its own brand and will continue to provide its own foods, coaching program and platforms.

HMR's meal replacement strategy takes away the struggles involved in making the right food choices to lose weight – and most people fail when they are left to their own devices when it comes to choosing to eat healthy. HMR meals are combined with fruits and vegetables to replace high-calorie foods and to create more filling and nutritious meals. Ten to 20 minutes of light, daily physical activity is also required to achieve weight-loss goals and maintain a healthy weight long-term.

HMR meal replacements include low-calorie shakes, meals, nutrition bars, and multigrain hot cereal.

While following the HMR diet, you can expect to feel hungry when first starting, but most report that the hunger goes away.

How the HMR Diet Works: Basics and Principles

The HMR diet works by putting your body in a calorie deficit by providing HMR shakes, HMR entrees, HMR bars, and other healthy snacks to help you reduce your calorie intake. A calorie deficit is when you are consuming less calories than you are burning. In order to get the energy that it needs, your body will burn stored fat which will result in weight loss.

The HMR diet tackles a typical weight loss problem. After going on a diet, many people rapidly gain weight back. Regaining weight is a result of your body's reference point. If you have carried extra weight for an extended period, your body will try to return to that weight.

HMR health coaches provide support through dedicated coaching groups and a free HMR app, which integrates with the HMR program website, including a custom online dashboard and other resources throughout.

Members develop regular physical activity routines with feedback from coaches and practice healthy dietary skills.

Physical activity gradually increases toward burning at least 2,000 calories weekly. Walking is a favorite.

There are two phases to the diet. Phase 1 focuses on weight loss with HMR meal replacements, while phase 2 focuses on weight maintenance through healthy lifestyle behaviors and habits.

Note: *While following the HMR diet, you can expect to feel hungry when first starting, but most report that the hunger goes away.*

Can I Lose Weight on the HMR Program?

Any diet may help you lose weight, but people who change their lifestyle through the HMR program can maintain significant weight loss through either the in-clinic (with or without medical supervision) or at-home options. HMR also offers a low-calorie diet plan, under medical supervision.

Losing weight can be simpler if you outsource meal preparation and limit food decisions and high-calorie temptations. In phase 1, HMR delivers all your low-calorie, heat-and-eat entrees and add-water-and-blend shakes. Sticking with HMR selections, eating fresh produce and meeting the recommended levels of moderate exercise should lead to weight loss.

The at-home program reports an average loss of 13 to 20 pounds overall within 12 weeks, with higher numbers for people who take part in weekly Zoom group coaching.

Short-Term Weight Loss

HMR can lead to short-term weight loss.

HMR-sponsored research shows participants with obesity using HMR meal replacements plus fruits and vegetables lost nearly 29 pounds more than those who just received weight loss counseling over 24 weeks.

Other HMR-sponsored research shows similar or better results. In one study, participants lost an average of 37.5 pounds in 18 weeks, and medically supervised patients lost 43.5 pounds in 19 weeks.

In a review of 39 randomly-controlled trials of commercial weight loss programs, participants in "very-low-calorie programs," including the HMR diet, lost 4% more weight in the short term than counseling, but longer-term results were mixed.

Long-Term Weight Loss

Its phase 2 is designed to promote healthy and sustainable weight loss over a longer period of time by helping people establish healthy eating and lifestyle habits.

Weight Maintenance and Management

Reviews of various conventional diets suggest that meal replacement strategies can safely and effectively lead to significant and sustainable weight loss.

HMR Program Options

HMR At-Home Program – Healthy Solutions Diet

This is HMR's most popular program option and involves two phases, with an average of 1,200 to 1,500 calories per day.

Phase One or the Quick Start Phase. The goal during this phase is to lose weight quickly. After your first three-week supply, you will receive HMR meals every two weeks; you will provide the fruits and vegetables yourself.

Phase Two or the Transition Phase. During this phase, you will maintain your target weight or continue losing weight at your own pace with the help of monthly HMR food deliveries combined with healthy food options and lifestyle changes. You will also receive coaching from dietitians and exercise physiologists through weekly phone calls.

In-Clinic Option

HMR clinic programs are offered by about 60 hospitals, medical practices, and other facilities throughout the U.S. The In-Clinic Option also combines the structured diet plan, healthy lifestyle strategies, and group support.

Prior to beginning any HMR program, you will undergo medical screening. Your overall assessment – which includes your health profile, medical history, and preferred diet – will determine whether or not your plan will be medically supervised, which will fall under the Decision-Free Diet plan.

Medically Supervised Decision-Free Diet Option

Individuals who need to lose 50 pounds or more are encouraged to follow the HMR Decision-Free plan. With only 500 to 1,000 calories per day, this option includes medical supervision. To stay within the extremely low-calorie requirement, only HMR meals are included in the diet; even the fruits and vegetables are excluded.

The HMR Healthy Solutions diet may also require medical supervision if the participant is also undergoing diabetes management through medications, or has another health condition that would require even closer monitoring on a restricted diet.

HMR Program Foods

Here's a list of some of the foods included in the HMR replacement meal plans. It's easy to create a wide variety of meals using HMR foods and HMR-approved recipes.

• HMR Multigrain Hot Cereal includes oats, wheat, corn, red currants, cranberries, and apple bits.

• HMR Savory Chicken entree, which you can toss into a green salad with a healthy vinaigrette dressing.

• HMR Shakes, which you can modify and blend with different kinds of fruits to create more enjoyable beverages and desserts.

• HMR Cheese and Basil Ravioli entree, which you can turn into a fuller meal with some steamed vegetables and a side of fresh vegetable salad.

• HMR Vegetarian Thai Curry with Brown Rice entree, which you can mix and match with a variety of vegetables to make a complete and palatable meal.

• HMR Chicken Enchilada entree.

• HMR Chicken Creole entree.

• HMR Chicken with Barbecue Sauce entree

• HMR Turkey Chili entree.

• HMR Chicken Pasta Parmesan entree.

• HMR 500 Chicken Soup, which you can enjoy on its own or mixed with another HMR chicken entree or your choice of vegetables.

• HMR Mushroom Risotto entree.

• HMR Five-Bean Casserole entree.

What Are the Health Benefits of the HMR Diet?

There are many health benefits to completing the HMR diet such as improved blood sugar, blood pressure, and cholesterol levels as well as weight loss and better nutritional awareness.

Improve blood sugar, blood pressure, and good cholesterol levels: HMR diet incorporates HMR shakes and HMR entrees for breakfast and lunch, which are low in sugar and sodium. HMR meal items are also low in fat and have no trans fats, which helps keep your cholesterol levels healthy.

Losing weight: HMR diet helps you lose weight quickly. HMR meals are low-calorie and convenient, which makes it easier to stick to the diet and stay within the calorie deficit. Losing weight is the primary benefit of the HMR diet.

Better nutrition and portion control: The HMR diet helps you learn proper portion sizes and nutrition. Knowing the appropriate portion size is one of the biggest challenges of maintaining a healthy weight.

What Are the Health Risks of the HMR Diet?

Like any diet, there are some negatives to the HMR diet such as lower metabolism, increased risk of bone loss, fertility and immunity issues.

Lower your metabolism – Another problem with staying at a calorie deficit for an extended time is that your body's metabolism can slow down. A slower metabolism can make it harder for your body to lose weight because you burn fewer calories.

Increase the risk of bone loss – The HMR diet can help you lose weight quickly, but it is vital to consider the potential health risks. Ensure you get enough calcium and vitamin D to maintain good bone health.

Fertility and immunity issues – Since you are at a severe calorie deficit, your body is not getting enough calories to complete all of its functions, including fertility and immunity. While on this diet, your body cannot protect itself against disease. You should also avoid trying to get pregnant while on this diet because the calorie deficit can negatively impact the fetus.

2

GETTING STARTED WITH THE HMR DIET

What Does the HMR Program Cost?

The first two-week Starter Kit retail cost is $221, but as of July 2023, there is a promotion for $50 off. This includes two canisters of HMR shakes, 28 HMR entrees, support materials, weekly group coaching and free shipping.

• There are no start-up or ongoing membership fees.

• The standard two-week reorder kits cost about $209.45, or about $15 a day, and includes Zoom group coaching and two weeks' worth of breakfasts, lunches, dinners and snacks – just add fruits and vegetables.

• You'll save on costs in the meat and processed-food sections of your grocery store, and on eating out, while possibly spending more money than you're used to spending in the produce aisle.

What Costs Are Related to the HMR Program?

HMR foods and outside groceries make up the bulk of your program expenses.

Doing HMR Program on a Budget

You can cut costs on HMR by taking simple steps:

• Take advantage of the special introductory prices.

• Look for grocery store sales on fresh fruits or vegetables.

• Choose less expensive canned or frozen produce.

Is HMR Program Easy to Follow?

High-touch, expert coaching for guidance, accountability and support is provided throughout both phases of the program, HMR representatives emphasize.

With the meals and shake mixes delivered right to your door, HMR phase 1 saves a lot of time at the supermarket, though you'll be frequenting the produce section and picking up allowed add-ins, such as diet sodas, vanilla extract, sugar-free gelatin mix, mustard, salsa and spices.

Because shakes made in a blender are more filling, you might want to consider bringing a blender to work or blending shakes at home and using a thermos for transport. Entrees and hot cereals are microwaveable, and packages are shelf-ready (no need to refrigerate).

There are resources for recipes. The 76-page recipe book in the HMR starter kit includes recipes for vanilla and chocolate-mix shakes, fruit smoothies, floats, ice cream, hot drinks and puddings, along with several recipes for HMR Multigrain Hot Cereal and HMR 500 Chicken Soup. Dozens of entrée-based recipes in the booklet include stroganoff Florentine, fajita bowl, BBQ sweet and sour chicken, pasta with spinach Alfredo sauce and shepherd's pie. For more options, you can turn to the HMR's website for hundreds of additional recipes.

Having entrees and shakes delivered to your door – with the option to also order foods like HMR Bars, chicken soup and multigrain cereals – should cut time at the grocery store. You won't have to spend much time meal planning, either, especially during phase 1.

Feeling full shouldn't be a problem. With six total meal and snack breaks throughout the day, not to mention the "more is better" option to add additional HMR foods if you're still hungry, you should feel as full as you need to. The phase 1 booklet says that, depending on someone's weight, a person would have to eat between eight and 10 shakes daily to stop losing weight. However, moderation is still a good idea with whatever diet you follow.

Who Should Not Try the HMR Program?

HMR lists certain circumstances in which people should not participate in its remote programs. These include:

• Pregnancy.

• Breastfeeding (in some cases).

• Active eating disorders.

• Allergies to milk protein, egg or corn.

• Having had bariatric (weight-loss) surgery within the past year.

• Under 18 years of age.

• Medical conditions such as advanced liver, kidney or heart disease.

• Currently receiving obesity treatments, such as nerve stimulation therapy, aspiration pump therapy or placement of an intragastric stomach balloon.

Does the HMR Program Work?

Subscribing to a meal replacement program or weight-loss meal delivery program is usually an effective way to lose excess weight. Most of the time, people who want to lose weight fail in their efforts to limit their food options and resist temptations. HMR's meal replacements, combined with the program's training and education to learn healthy lifestyle strategies and its support system, do help participants achieve weight loss.

The HMR program requires minimum effort on the part of the participants. As long as you stick to the recommended HMR diet plan and engage in adequate physical activity, you can experience significant weight loss and sustain it until you reach your target weight.

However, given the plan's highly restrictive structure, it may be difficult to commit to long enough to attain one's weight-loss goal or to maintain it.

3

THE HMR DIET PLAN IN DETAIL

Phase 1: Weight Loss Diet

In the initial weight loss phase, program members can lose weight quickly by following HMR's clinically validated weight loss plan with the help of coaching and online support. Members follow a structured, high-volume diet, using a full line of HMR foods – with or without fruits and vegetables, depending on the diet plan. The structured, meal replacement-based diet reduces decisions, allowing members to take a break from current food routines. They also begin to incorporate short bouts of physical activity into their lifestyle.

HMR recommends committing to phase 1 for at least eight weeks. Expected weight loss is 1 to 2 pounds per week, with an average weight loss of 23 pounds over the first 12 weeks.

The daily diet plan for phase 1 includes these three components:

Three HMR shakes.

Two HMR entrees.

Five full-cup servings of fruits and vegetables.

If you're hungry, you can eat more of these lower-calorie fruits and vegetables and still lose weight. For variety, you can mix and match HMR foods and the produce you buy. You're urged to eat often and always have food with you to avoid temptations. You'll learn strategies for handling social situations and activities that center around food.

Phase 2: Weight Maintenance

In phase 2, you'll start to cut back on HMR foods as you introduce other healthy foods, primarily lots of lean proteins, whole grains, fruits and vegetables, dairy and healthy fats. You'll focus more on establishing healthy lifestyle habits, such as regular physical activity, while maintaining your phase 1 weight loss or continuing to lose weight at your own pace. Weekly virtual group coaching sessions with an HMR coach are available throughout for support and to encourage accountability.

As the food plan shifts, you'll eat some HMR foods and continue 35 servings of fruits and vegetables a week, gradually adding in healthy non-HMR, low-calorie foods. You begin making food choices while strategically using at least 14 HMR foods a week. You'll focus on lean proteins, using low-calorie cooking methods, such as baking, broiling and steaming, and including grains, and you'll practice balancing low- and higher-calorie days along with physical activity levels.

Physical Activity

During both phases of the diet, you'll incorporate exercise and physical activity into your daily routine. The goal is to burn at least 2,000 calories or more with physical activity each week. Strategies include spreading out activity in short amounts throughout the day and doing moderate-intensity exercise, such as walking, swimming, dancing or using a treadmill at a moderate pace.

Physical activity lowers your risk of heart disease and diabetes, helps keep weight off and increases your energy level. Most experts suggest getting at least 30 minutes of moderate-intensity exercise – like brisk walking – most or all days of the week.

Tracking

The free HMR mobile app allows users to track their physical activity and food intake to ensure they stay accountable.

Further Details on the HMR Diet Plan

How Much Should You Exercise on the HMR Diet?

HMR encourages moderate exercise, such as walking briskly, swimming, or dancing. You can tailor this to your schedule. For example, you might take a 10- to 20-minute walk after breakfast, lunch, and dinner; or plan a few longer walks every week.

The HMR program recommends walking every day during the first week to build the habit. Your goal is to burn 2,000 calories through physical activity weekly.[7] Remember that this is a lower-calorie diet, and you should talk to your doctor if you are planning vigorous exercise while restricting calories. Also, be sure to increase exercise slowly, especially if you are new to a workout program.

How to Do HMR Diet?

The HMR diet is easy to start and follow. You can begin the diet by visiting the HMR website and purchasing your desired plan. After paying, you will receive your prepackaged smoothies, bars, and meals. You will also receive an HMR lifestyle guide to help you stay on track.

In addition to prepackaged meals, you can supplement your food with fresh fruits and vegetables. You need to follow the diet for the recommended time and exercise if you want to achieve your weightloss goals.

While on the HMR diet, you will consume 1200-1400 calories daily. At this level of consumption, you will be at a 600-1000 calorie deficit.

The first phase of the HMR diet can last 8-12 weeks, depending on how much weight you want to lose. The second phase can last up to four weeks for a total of 12-16 weeks.

While completing the HMR diet, you should exercise regularly, drink lots of water, and get enough sleep. Exercise helps to boost your metabolism and burn more calories while also helping you stay motivated.

What Are the Foods That You Can Eat While on an HMR Diet?

While on the HMR diet, you should avoid almost all foods since you consume prepackaged meals. However you can eat fresh fruits and vegetables.

• **Fruits**: apples, oranges, bananas, and berries

• **Vegetables**: celery, carrots, and broccoli

• **Grains**: You cannot eat any additional grains besides what is included in the HMR meals.

• **Legumes**: Legumes are high calorie and you cannot eat them.

• **Nuts**: Nuts are another high calorie food you should avoid.

• **Seeds**: You cannot eat seeds on the HMR diet.

• **Healthy fats**: No healthy fats are allowed on this diet.

• **Proteins**: The only proteins you can eat are the ones provided in the meal plan.

What Are the Foods That You Should Avoid While on an HMR Diet?

Since the HMR diet focuses on prepacked meals, you should avoid any foods not included in your meal plan.

• **Meat**: steak, pork, bacon

• **Poultry**: chicken and turkey

• **Fish and shellfish**: canned tuna

• **Meat-based ingredients**: deli meats

• **Eggs**: boiled or fried eggs

• **Dairy products**: sour cream, yogurt, and milk

You need to avoid these foods because they will increase your calorie intake and take you out of a calorie deficit. Getting out of a calorie deficit will prevent you from losing weight.

Who Should Do the HMR Diet?

People whose primary goal is losing weight should do the HMR diet. The focus of this diet is to put you in a calorie deficit to help you lose weight and establish a new body reference point. It can also be an ideal diet for bodybuilders preparing for a competition. A large calorie deficit can help you develop a lot of body definition.

What Is a Sample HMR Diet Plan?

A sample meal plan from HMR includes three HMR shakes and one HMR Entree. For breakfast, you can have an HMR shake with 1/2 cup of berries or an HMR Entrée with a salad. You can have an HMR shake and HMR Entrée or HMR Nutri-Bar for lunch. You can have an HMR shake and HMR Entrée or HMR Nutri-Bar for dinner. You will repeat this process for the entire first phase of the diet program.

What Are the Best Recipes for HMR Diet?

It is important to remember that you do not need recipes during the first phase of the HMR diet. During the second phase, these are some of the best recipes you can incorporate.

• **Crispy Veggies**: This vegetable dish will make it easy to get in your daily vegetable servings while also holding off your cravings.

• **Risotto Riot**: The combination of fresh vegetables and risotto is filling and delicious.

• **Healthy Turkey Burgers**: Substituting turkey for beef cuts down the number of calories.

• **Spiced Carrot and Lentil Soup**: This tasty soup will keep you warm and full even on a cold night while dieting.

• **Sesame Beef with Noodles**: This beef and noodle dish is filled with protein which will help you avoid hunger pains.

What Are the Facts About the HMR Diet?

There are some important facts you should know about the HMR diet including what happens during the first week, the cost, how it compares to the Atkins diet, and the weight loss.

• **Research based**: The HMR diet is a safe and tested method for losing weight. Many scientific studies have proven HMR to be an effective way of losing weight.

• **The First Week**: During the first week of the HMR diet, you will have low energy levels and may be irritable due to the caloric restrictions. These symptoms will subside over time.

• **The Cost**: The HMR Diet is $90-110 per week. The price depends on what package you select.

• **Comparison with Atkins Diet**: The HMR and Atkins diet are similar because they both provide flexible pre-packaged meals delivered to your door.

• **Weight Loss:** The HMR diet can be an excellent way for most people to lose weight and establish healthier eating habits. By following the HMR diet, you can learn how to make better food choices that will lead to long-term weight loss.

HMR Diet Food Menu and Sample Shopping List

During the initial weight loss phase of the HMR diet, you do not need to do much food shopping, preparation, or cooking. You will order a specific amount of HMR-approved foods, which will be shipped to your house. The only other foods you will purchase on your own are fruits and vegetables. Here are some of the produce you can choose from, according to HMR:

• Lettuce

• Spinach

• Kale

• Tomatoes

• Green beans

- Brussels sprouts

- Broccoli

- Cauliflower

- Zucchini

- Eggplant

- Carrots

- Peppers

- Oranges

- Berries (strawberries, blueberries, raspberries)

- Melon

- Apples

- Kiwi

• Pears

• Pineapple

• Mango

A Sample Menu on the HMR Diet

All the food in the initial phase will be HMR-approved (see the complete food list below). You're encouraged to consume at least three shakes, two entrées, and five servings of fruits and vegetables each day. If you are still hungry, you can eat more HMR food or pump up the volume of your meals with additional vegetables alongside the entrées or extra fruit in your shake.

Breakfast: Multigrain hot cereal with 1 cup of fruit

Snack: Chocolate shake

Lunch: Penne pasta with meatballs and 2 cups of vegetables

Snack: 1 cup of fruit

Dinner: Fiesta chicken and 2 cups of vegetables

Dessert: Vanilla shake with 1 cup of frozen fruit

A Complete HMR Diet Food List

HMR food is all packaged and shelf-stable. Here's what is offered, according to its website:

• Shake mixes

• Multigrain hot cereal

• Chicken soup

• Bars (fudge graham bar, chocolate peanut butter, double chocolate chip, iced oatmeal, lemon)

Entrées

• Beef stroganoff

• Cheese and basil ravioli

• Chicken enchiladas

• Chicken pasta parmesan

• Chicken with barbecue sauce

• Crustless chicken pot pie

• Fiesta chicken

• Lasagna with meat sauce

• Mac and cheese

• Mushroom risotto

• Pasta fagioli

- Penne pasta with meatballs

- Rotini chicken Alfredo

- Sausage and potato in gravy

- Turkey chili with beans

- Vegetable stew with beef

- Whole-grain medley with chicken

4

HMR DIET RECIPES YOU MUST TRY!

DELIGHTFUL RECIPES FOR BREAKFAST

Chicken Mini Frittatas

Ingredients

• 1 pound skinless boneless chicken breast

• 2 medium eggs

• ½ cup almond flour

• 1 cup shredded mozzarella cheese

• 2 tablespoons finely chopped fresh basil

• 2 tablespoons chopped chives

• 2 tablespoons chopped parsley

• ½ teaspoon garlic powder

• Sea salt and black pepper, to taste

• 1 tablespoon olive oil Ranch dressing, for serving

Instructions

1. Chop the uncooked chicken breast into tiny pieces, and then place the pieces in a large mixing bowl.

2. Stir in the almond flour, eggs, mozzarella, basil, chives, parsley, garlic powder, salt, and pepper. Mix well to combine.

3. Add the oil to a large nonstick pan and heat over medium-low heat. Scoop the chicken mixture into the pan, then slightly flatten to create a frittata. Cook the frittatas in batches, about 4 per batch.

4. Fry at medium-low temperature until golden brown on both sides, about 6–8 minutes.

5. Serve with ranch dressing.

Spinach Fritters

Ingredients

• 1 tablespoon + 2 teaspoons extra-virgin olive oil, divided

• 1 cup diced potatoes

• 1 medium onion, diced

- 1 garlic clove, minced

- ½ cup spinach leaves

- 1 ⅓ cups chickpea flour

- 2 large eggs, lightly beaten

- ½ cup water

- ½ teaspoon salt

Instructions

1. Heat 1 tablespoon of olive oil in a non-stick frying pan over medium-high heat. Stir in the diced potatoes and cook for 10 minutes, until they are lightly golden and start to soften.

2. Add the onion, garlic, and remaining 2 teaspoons of olive oil. Cook for another 5 minutes, stirring occasionally, until the onions soften.

3. Add the spinach and cook for 2 minutes, until the spinach wilts.

4. Whisk together the chickpea flour, eggs, water, and salt in a medium bowl. Pour the mixture into the pan and mix well, until the potatoes are coated with the mixture.

5. Decrease the heat to medium-low and cook for 5–7 minutes, until golden. Flip and cook for another 5 minutes, until golden. Remove from the heat.

6. Serve and enjoy! Refrigerate leftovers in an airtight container for up to 3 days.

Tunisian Shakshuka

Ingredients

• 2 tablespoons extra-virgin olive oil

- 1 onion, minced

- 2 red bell peppers, diced

- 2 garlic cloves, chopped

- 1 (15-ounce) can diced tomatoes

- 1 teaspoon spicy harissa

- 1 teaspoon salt

- 1 teaspoon black pepper

- 4 medium eggs

- 1 tablespoon chopped parsley

Instructions

1. Heat the olive oil in a heavy cast-iron skillet over medium heat.

2. Add the onion and bell peppers and cook, stirring occasionally, until soft, about 5 minutes.

3. Stir in the garlic and cook for 1 minute. Stir in the tomatoes and harissa and cook, stirring, for 7 minutes.

4. Season with salt and pepper and add more harissa, if desired.

5. Make 4 holes in the tomato mixture with the back of a wooden spoon and crack an egg into each hole.

6. Cover the skillet and cook for 3–4 minutes, until the egg whites firm.

7. Sprinkle with fresh parsley and serve with pita or crusty bread, if desired.

Zucchini, Pea, & Halloumi Fritters

Ingredients

• 3 medium zucchinis, grated

• 1 cup coarsely grated Halloumi

• 1 cup almond flour

• ½ cup frozen peas

• ¼ cup chopped fresh dill or mint

• 2 eggs, lightly beaten

• 1 ½ teaspoons Himalayan salt

• ½ teaspoon ground black pepper

• 3 tablespoons extra-virgin olive oil

Instructions

1. Combine the zucchini, Halloumi, almond flour, peas, dill or mint, eggs, salt, and black pepper in amedium bowl and mix well.

2. Place the olive oil in a large frying pan overmedium-high heat.

3. Spoon about 3 tablespoons of the batter per pancake into the frying pan and flatten slightlyusing a spatula.

4. Cook the pancakes for 3–4 minutes each, flipping halfway through, until golden. Placethem onto paper towels to drain.

5. Repeat steps 3–4 until all the batter has been used.

6. Serve warm. Refrigerate leftovers in an airtight container for up to 3 days.

Simple Cheese & Veggie Omelet

Ingredients

- 4 large eggs

- 2 tablespoons almond milk

- 1 teaspoon Himalayan salt

- ½ teaspoon ground black pepper

- ½ teaspoon Spanish paprika

- ¼ teaspoon ground allspice

- ¼ teaspoon baking powder

- 1 ½ teaspoons extra-virgin olive oil

- 3 tablespoons chopped fresh parsley

- 3 tablespoons chopped fresh mint

• 1⁄2 cup halved cherry tomatoes (optional)

• 2 tablespoons sliced and pitted Kalamata olives (optional)

• 1⁄4–1⁄3 cup drained and quartered marinated artichoke hearts(optional)

• 2–4 tablespoons crumbled feta cheese, as desired (optional)

Instructions

1. Whisk together the eggs, almond milk, salt,pepper, paprika, allspice, and baking powder inmedium bowl.

2. Heat the olive oil in a 10-inch skillet overmedium-high heat. Tilt the skillet so the oil fullycoats the bottom.

3. Pour the egg mixture into the skillet and stir itquickly with a spatula for 5 seconds. Push thecooked bits of the egg toward the center of thepan while tilting the pan to allow the raw egg tofill the empty spaces.

4. Cook the omelet for 1–2 minutes, until thebottom is golden and the eggs are nearly set, thenremove from the heat. Add the toppings of yourchoice to one side of the omelet and fold over theempty side onto the toppings.

5. Slice the omelet in half, place each half on aserving plate, and sprinkle with parsley and mint, if desired.

Overnight Cereal in a Jar

Ingredients

• ⅔ cup almond milk

• ½ cup shelled hemp hearts

• 2 tablespoons chia seeds

• 2 teaspoons erythritol sweetener (such as Swerve)

• 1 teaspoon vanilla extract Berries, sugar-free chocolate chips, nuts, nut butter, and/ or Greek yogurt, for topping (optional)

Instructions

1. Combine the almond milk, hemp hearts, chia seeds, sweetener, and vanilla in a bowl. Cover with a lid or plastic wrap and place in the refrigerator to chill for at least 6 hours, or overnight.

2. In the morning, add any desired toppings, such as berries, sugar-free chocolate chips, or nuts for

added texture, a tablespoon of nut butter for flavor, or full-fat Greek yogurt for creaminess.

Pistachio & Grape Yogurt Bowl

Ingredients

- 3 cups purple grapes

- 2 cups whole-fat or 2% Greek yogurt

- 1/4 cup chopped pistachios

- 1/4 cup chopped fresh mint

- 1/4 cup honey

- Juice of 1/2 lemon

- 2 tablespoons granola

- 2 tablespoons chopped walnuts

Instructions

1. Combine the grapes, yogurt, pistachios, mint, honey, and lemon juice in a food processor or blender and mix until smooth.

2. Divide the mixture among four serving cups or dishes and garnish with walnuts and granola, if desired.

Cinnamon Roll Porridge With Cranberries

Ingredients

• 1 cup non-dairy milk

• ½ cup gluten-free quick oats

• 1 banana, mashed, plus ¼ banana, sliced

• 1 teaspoon ground cardamom

• 1 teaspoon raw honey

• 1/4 cup dried cranberries

• 1 teaspoon ground cinnamon

• 2 tablespoons almond butter

Instructions

1. Combine the milk, oats, mashed banana, cardamom, and honey in a small saucepan over medium-high heat. Cook for 5 minutes, stirring occasionally, until it thickens.

2. Transfer to a small heat-safe bowl, add the cranberries and cinnamon, and mix until well combined.

3. Top with the almond butter and banana slices. Serve immediately or refrigerate for the next day and serve cold.

Cauliflower and Egg Salad

Ingredients

- 1½ cups vegetable stock

- 2 cups fresh cauliflower florets

- 4 hard-boiled eggs, peeled and cubed

- ¼ cup cherry tomatoes

- 2 tablespoons chopped fresh parsley

- 2 tablespoons chopped green onion

- ½ cup heavy cream

- 2 tablespoons light mayonnaise

- 1 tablespoon vinegar

- 1 teaspoon extra-virgin olive oil

• 4 black olives, sliced

Instructions

1. Pour the vegetable stock into an Instant Pot and insert the steamer basket.

2. Place the cauliflower florets in the steamer basket, seal the pot with the lid, and cook the cauliflower on high for 14 minutes.

3. Allow the pressure to release naturally for 4 minutes, then use the quick-release function and remove the lid.

4. Place the cauliflower florets in a large bowl. Add the hard-boiled eggs, cherry tomatoes, parsley, green onion, heavy cream, mayonnaise, vinegar, and olive oil, stirring to combine.

5. Garnish with black olives and divide among four serving bowls. Refrigerate leftovers in an airtight container for up to 3 days.

Golden Shrimp & Avocado Toast

Ingredients

• 1 pound shrimp, raw

• Juice of 2 limes, divided

• 1 teaspoon smoked paprika

• ½ teaspoon kosher salt

• ¼ teaspoon cayenne pepper

• 4 slices whole-wheat bread, toasted

• 4 large avocados, sliced

• 1⁄2 large tomato, chopped

• 1⁄4 cup chopped fresh cilantro, optional

Instructions

1. Combine the shrimp, juice of 1 lime, smoked paprika, salt, and cayenne pepper in a medium bowl, tossing to combine. Cover the bowl with a dishtowel or plastic wrap and refrigerate for 15–20 minutes to marinate.

2. Turn your grill to high. Arrange the shrimp on the grill and cook for 3–4 minutes, until golden.

3. Place the toast slices on a platter, then arrange the avocado slices on the toast. Top with the shrimp and garnish with the remaining lime juice, the tomatoes, and cilantro, if desired. Serve warm.

Raspberry and Granola Greek Yogurt

Ingredients

- ½ cup sugar-free, gluten-free granola

- ¼ cup fresh raspberries

- 1 teaspoon chia seeds

- 1 teaspoon roasted pumpkin seeds

- 1 teaspoon toasted sesame seeds

- ⅔ cup plain Greek yogurt

- 1 tablespoon maple syrup

- ½ teaspoon ground cinnamon

Instructions

1. In an 8-ounce container, combine the granola, raspberries, chia seeds, pumpkin seeds, sesame seeds, Greek yogurt, and maple syrup.

2. Sprinkle the ground cinnamon on top of the granola-yogurt mixture.

3. Cover and refrigerate for 1 hour to chill, then serve.

Tangy Tuna Sandwich

Ingredients

• 2 (5-oz.) cans tuna in oil, drained

• 5 pickles, thinly sliced

• ½ apple, thinly sliced

• ½ cup light mayonnaise

- ¼ cup fresh cilantro, chopped

- 3 tablespoons thinly sliced chives

- 1 tablespoon Dijon mustard

- 1 tablespoon unsalted butter

- 6 slices gluten-free bread, toasted

- 1 medium tomato, sliced

- ½ cucumber, sliced

Instructions

1. Combine the tuna, pickles, apple, mayonnaise, cilantro, chives, and Dijon mustard in a medium bowl, mixing well, until thoroughly combined.

2. Spread the butter onto the toasted bread slices and top three with the tuna mixture, tomato slices,

and cucumber slices. Finish by placing the remaining buttered slices on top and serve.

Greek Vegetable Omelet

Ingredients

• 4 large eggs

• 2 tablespoons fat-free milk

• ½ teaspoon paprika

• ¼ teaspoon allspice

• ½ teaspoon salt

• ½ teaspoon black pepper

• 1½ teaspoons extra-virgin olive oil

• ½ cup crumbled feta cheese

- ½ cup halved cherry tomatoes

- ⅓ cup drained marinated artichoke hearts

- 3 tablespoons chopped fresh parsley

- 3 tablespoons chopped fresh mint

- 2 tablespoons pitted kalamata olives

Instructions

1. In a medium bowl, whisk together all the omelet Ingredients except the olive oil.

2. Coat a 10-inch nonstick skillet with the olive oil and set it over medium-high heat.

3. Once the oil is shimmering, pour the egg mixture into the skillet and stir it with a spatula for 5 seconds.

4. Push the cooked egg in from the edge of the skillet to the center and tilt the pan to allow the uncooked egg to fill in the empty spots.

5. Cook the omelet for 1 minute, until the eggs are set, then remove it from the heat. Spoon your desired add-ons onto one side of the omelet and use a spatula to fold the remaining half of the omelet over the add-ons.

6. Slice the omelet into two portions. Serve with warm pita bread, if desired.

Breakfast Potato Salad

Ingredients

- 1½ cups water

- 2 pounds baby red potatoes, peeled and quartered

- 1/4 cup balsamic vinegar

- 1/4 cup extra-virgin olive oil

- 1 small onion, chopped

- 2 teaspoons chopped parsley

- 1 teaspoon chopped thyme

- 1 teaspoon salt

- 1/2 teaspoon ground black pepper

Instructions

1. Place the water into an Instant Pot, then insert the steamer basket. Add the baby potatoes to the steamer basket.

2. Set the Instant Pot to non-venting, seal with the lid, and cook the potatoes on high for 12 minutes, until tender.

3. Switch to venting and allow the pressure to release naturally for 10 minutes, then switch to the quick-release function.

4. Remove the lid and place the potatoes into a large mixing bowl. Add the balsamic vinegar, olive oil, onion, parsley, thyme, salt, and pepper, tossing to combine. Divide among four serving bowls.

5. Refrigerate leftovers in an airtight container for up to 3 days.

Almond Flour Pancakes

Ingredients

- 1 heaping cup finely ground almond flour

- 2 tablespoons erythritol sweetener (such as Swerve)

- 1 teaspoon baking powder

- ⅛ teaspoon salt

- 2 large eggs

- ⅓ cup unsweetened coconut milk

- 1 tablespoon coconut oil

- ½ teaspoon vanilla extract

- Unsalted butter, for frying

Instructions

1. Combine all the Ingredients in a large bowl and mix well to form a smooth batter.

2. Heat a large skillet over medium-low heat and add ½ teaspoon of butter. When the butter is melted, drop ¼ cup batter onto the pan for each pancake. Cook until bubbles form around the

edges, then flip and cook for an additional 1–2 minutes, or until evenly browned.

3. Repeat with the remaining batter, adding more butter to the skillet as needed. You should end up with a total of 6–8 pancakes. Serve warm with butter and sugar-free syrup.

DELIGHTFUL RECIPES FOR LUNCH

Mediterranean Chicken Casserole

Ingredients

• 1 HMR Whole Grain Medley with Chicken entree

• 1/2 Cup canned artichoke hearts (in water), (drained and quartered)

• 1/2 Cup chickpeas (drained and rinsed)

• 1/2 Cup red bell pepper (diced)

• 1 Tbs lemon juice

• 1 Tbs non-fat sour cream

• 1 Tsp chopped garlic

• Salt and pepper to taste

Instructions

1. To enjoy cold- simply combine all Ingredients.

2. To enjoy hot- preheat oven to 350 degrees.

3. Place all Ingredients in a bowl and mix to combine.

4. Spray an oven-safe dish with non-stick cooking spray, add the combined Ingredients, and bake uncovered for about 25 min.

Risotto Peanut Lettuce Wraps

• 1/2 cup carrots (diced)

• 1/2 cup purple cabbage (chopped)

• 1 HMR Mushroom Risotto Entree

• 1/2 cup water chestnuts (diced)

• 1 Tbsp. low-sodium soy sauce

• 1 Tbsp. PB2 Powdered Peanut Butter

• 4 leaves romaine lettuce

Instructions

1. Place a skillet over medium heat and spray with cooking spray. Saute carrots and cabbage until tender.

2. Add entree and water chestnuts to vegetables and cook until warm.

3. Stir in soy sauce and PB2.

4. Spoon into romaine lettuce leaves and roll.

Roasted Veggie Mac and Cheese

Ingredients

• 1 HMR Creamy Mac & Cheese Entree

• 1/2 cup brussel sprouts

• 1/2 cup cubed sweet potato

• 1/2 cup chopped cauliflower

• 1/2 cup chopped broccoli

• Dash of salt and pepper

Instructions

1. Preheat oven to 350 degrees.

2. Place vegetables on a baking sheet, sprinkle with salt and pepper, and bake for 30 minutes or until tender.

3. Heat entree according to package and mix with roasted vegetables.

Garlic Shrimp

Ingredients

- 1 pound shrimp, peeled and deveined

- 1 teaspoon salt

- 1 teaspoon pepper

- 3 tablespoons butter, divided

- 1 tablespoon olive oil

- 4 garlic cloves, minced

- 1 teaspoon paprika

- ¼ cup fumet

- 1 tablespoon sriracha

- 1 teaspoon crushed red pepper flakes

- 1 tablespoon lemon juice

- 1 tablespoon fresh chopped parsley or cilantro

Instructions

1. Season the shrimp with the salt and pepper and set aside. Place a large nonstick skillet over medium heat and add 1 tablespoon of butter and the olive oil. Add the shrimp and sauté 1 minute. Add the minced garlic and paprika to the shrimp, stir to combine, and cook the shrimp for 1 minute. Then add the fumet and sriracha. Reduce the sauce for 1 minute, making sure not to overcook the shrimp.

2. Pour 1 tablespoon of the lemon juice over the top of the cooked shrimp. Remove the shrimp from heat, garnish with the parsley, lemon slices, and crushed red pepper. Serve with cauliflower rice or zucchini noodles.

Chicken Salad Wrap

Ingredients

• 1½ pounds cold cooked chicken

• ½ cup sour cream

• 5 tablespoons sugar-free mayonnaise

• 3 tablespoons lemon juice

• 1 stalk celery, finely chopped

• ⅓ cup chopped walnuts

• 2 teaspoons chopped chives

• ¼ teaspoon garlic powder

• 10 lettuce leaves

Instructions

1. Cube the chilled chicken and place in a large serving bowl. Add all the remaining Ingredients and stir until the chicken is fully coated.

2. Serve cold on the lettuce leaves or a wrap of your choice. Refrigerate and store for up to 3 days.

Chicken Soup

Ingredients

• 4 boneless, skinless chicken breasts

• 1½ cups chunky tomato salsa

• 2 cups chicken bone broth

• ½ pound Manchego cheese, cubed small

• 1 tablespoon chopped cilantro

• 1 cup julienned cabbage

• 2 tablespoons olive oil

• Salt and black pepper, to taste

• 1 small avocado, sliced

Instructions

1. In a pan, heat the olive oil and add the chicken pieces. Cook until golden brown.

2. Place the chicken, broth, and tomato salsa in a large pot, bring to a boil, and cook for 15 minutes. Add the cabbage and cilantro and cook for another 10 minutes at low temperature. Season with salt and pepper.

3. Remove from heat. Serve, garnishing with cheese cubes and avocado.

Chicken Souvlaki

Ingredients

• 4 boneless, skinless chicken breasts, cut into 1-inch cubes

• ⅓ cup extra-virgin olive oil

• 2 tablespoons lemon juice

• 3 garlic cloves, minced

• 2 teaspoons dried oregano

• 1 teaspoon dried parsley

• 1 teaspoon sea salt

• ½ teaspoon black pepper

• ½ cup tzatziki sauce, to serve

Instructions

1. Combine the chicken, olive oil, lemon juice, garlic, oregano, parsley, salt, and pepper in a bowl and toss to combine.

2. Cover with plastic wrap and chill for a minimum of 30 minutes.

3. Heat your grill to medium-high and thread the chicken onto skewers.

4. Grill the chicken skewers for 3–4 minutes per side, until cooked through.

5. Place the chicken on a serving platter along with tzatziki sauce and pita bread, if desired. Serve immediately.

Prosciutto and Pesto Sandwich

Ingredients

- 1 tablespoon pesto

- 1 loaf whole-wheat ciabatta bread

- ½ cup halved cherry tomatoes

- ½ cup drained artichoke hearts

- ½ cup prosciutto

- ½ cup arugula

Instructions

1. Cut the ciabatta bread in half horizontally, then spread ½ tablespoon of pesto onto the cut side of each half.

2. Layer the cherry tomatoes on the bottom half and top with the artichoke hearts, prosciutto, and arugula. Place the remaining half of the bread on top.

3. Push a wooden skewer into the sandwich to make it easier to eat. Serve and enjoy!

Salmon and Spinach Salad

Ingredients

• 2 tablespoons extra-virgin olive oil

• 2 (6-ounce) salmon fillets

• ½ teaspoon salt

• ¼ teaspoon black pepper

• 4 cups baby spinach

• 2 tomatoes, chopped

• 1 avocado, diced

• 1 cucumber, sliced

• ¼ cup chopped red onion

• 1 tablespoon capers, drained For the dressing Juice of 1 lemon

• 1 tablespoon extra-virgin olive oil

• ½ teaspoon salt

• ¼ tablespoon black pepper

Instructions

1. To make the salad, heat the olive oil in a skillet over medium-high heat.

2. Sprinkle the salmon fillets with the salt and pepper and add them to the skillet. Cook for 4–5 minutes on one side, then flip the salmon fillets over and cook for 3 minutes more, until the fish flakes easily with a fork. Remove from the heat and set aside.

3. Divide the baby spinach, tomatoes, avocado, cucumber, red onion, and capers between three serving bowls. Slice the salmon fillets and divide into three servings, topping the salad.

4. To make the dressing, whisk together all the Ingredients. Pour the dressing over the salmon before serving.

Chicken Wraps

Ingredients

- 6 large lettuce leaves (iceberg)

- 6 chicken tenders, grilled

- 6 slices bacon

- 6 slices ham

- 6 slices Monterey Jack cheese

- 6 slices tomatoes

- 6 slices avocado

- 1 carrot, julienned

- ¼ cup purple cabbage, julienned

- Salt and pepper, to taste

Instructions

1. Lay 1 lettuce leaf onto a plate and lay one piece each of ham, chicken, and cheese on top; then add tomato, avocado, carrot, and cabbage.

2. Wrap it up and use a toothpick to hold it closed, if necessary. Serve with ranch dressing or mayonnaise.

Chili

Ingredients

• 1 pound extra lean ground beef

• 1 bell pepper, chopped

• 1 small sweet onion, chopped

• 2 tablespoons garlic, minced

• 1 (8-ounce) can tomato sauce

- 1 (8-ounce) can crushed tomatoes

- 1 (4-ounce) can diced green chilis

- 2–3 tablespoons chili powder

- 1 teaspoon pink Himalayan salt

Instructions

1. Combine the ground beef, pink Himalayan salt, bell pepper, onions, and garlic in a medium soup pot and cook, stirring, until the beef is well browned, 10–13 minutes. Drain off the grease, then return the pot to the heat.

2. Add all the remaining Ingredients, starting with just 2 tablespoons of the chili powder, and stir to completely combine. Bring to a boil, then reduce the heat to low and simmer for 30 minutes.

3. Taste the chili and adjust the seasoning with the remaining tablespoon of chili powder as needed. Cook for 15–20 minutes more.

4. Serve hot. Store leftovers in the fridge in an airtight container for up to 3 days.

Avocado and Chickpea Salad

Ingredients

• 1 (15-ounce) can chickpeas, drained

• 1 large cucumber, sliced

• 1 cup whole cherry tomatoes

• 1 ripe avocado, sliced

• ¼ cup tightly packed fresh parsley leaves

• 1 tablespoon extra-virgin olive oil

- Juice of ½ large lemon

- Sea salt, to season

- Black pepper, to season

Instructions

1. Combine the chickpeas, cucumber, tomatoes, avocado, and parsley in a medium bowl.

2. Add the olive oil, lemon juice, salt, and black pepper to the salad mixture, stirring to Combine. Serve and enjoy!

Avocado Seafood Wraps

Ingredients

- 5 ounces shrimp, peeled and deveined

- 3 ounces crab meat,finely chopped

- $1/4$ cup heavy cream

- 1 teaspoon unsalted butter

- $3/4$ teaspoon ground coriander

- $1/2$ teaspoon ground cayenne pepper

- $1/4$ teaspoon minced garlic

- 2 tablespoons plain Greek yogurt

- 3 (8-inch) whole-wheat tortillas

- 1 avocado, sliced

- 1 cucumber, sliced

- 2 tablespoons parsley, optional

Instructions

1. Combine the shrimp, crab meat, heavy cream,butter, garlic, coriander, and cayenne pepper

in a large saucepan over medium-high heat. Cook for 5–6 minutes, stirring occasionally, until the shrimp is bright pink. Remove from the heat and set aside.

2. Spread the yogurt onto the tortillas.

3. Arrange the avocado and cucumber on the tortillas, then add the seafood mixture.

4. Roll the tortillas up over the filling, folding in the sides, and use a toothpick to prevent the filling from falling out. Serve immediately.

Orange & Pomegranate Salad

Ingredients

• 1 tablespoon extra-virgin olive oil

• 1 tablespoon honey

- Juice of 1 lime

- 1 1/2 teaspoons orange blossom water, optional

- 1 cup thinly sliced red onions

- 25 fresh mint leaves,chopped

- 6 navel oranges, peeled and sliced into rounds

- 1/8 teaspoon kosher salt

- 1/8 teaspoon sweet paprika

- 1/8 teaspoon ground cinnamon

- Seeds (arils) of 1 pomegranate

Instructions

1. Whisk together the olive oil, honey, lime juice, and orange blossom water, if using, in a small bowl and set aside.

2. Place the red onions into a small bowl of ice water and set aside for 5 minutes to allow their flavor to mellow. Drain the onions and dry thoroughly.

3. Arrange half of the mint leaves around the edge of a serving bowl.

4. Place the orange slices and onions in the bowl and sprinkle with the salt, paprika, and cinnamon.

5. Drizzle the dressing over the salad, add the pomegranate seeds and remaining mint leaves, and set aside for 5 minutes to allow the flavors to blend. Serve and enjoy!

Chili Nachos

Ingredients

• 3 cups keto tortilla chips

- 1 cup shredded cheddar cheese

- ½ cup leftover Chili (page 70), warmed

- ¼ cup salsa

- 2 tablespoons sour cream

- ½ avocado, chopped

- 1 small jalapeño, diced

Instructions

1. Preheat the oven to 375°F.

2. Spread the chips out on a baking sheet and sprinkle with the cheese. Bake until the cheese is melted and beginning to brown, 5–6 minutes.

3. Remove from the oven and transfer the chips to a serving plate. Top with warm chili. Garnish your

nachos with salsa, sour cream, avocado, and jalapeño, in whatever order makes you the happiest.

Pasta Frittata

Ingredients

• 1 cup whole milk

• 3 eggs, beaten

• 2 ounces cheddar cheese, shredded

• 1 teaspoon salt

• 1 teaspoon chopped fresh dill

• 1/4 teaspoon crushed red pepper flakes

• 1/4 teaspoon paprika

• 1/4 teaspoon ground black pepper

• 2 ounces cooked tagliatelle pasta or linguine pasta (follow package Instructions and cook to al dente)

• 1 teaspoon extra-virgin olive oil

Instructions

1. Preheat the oven to 360°F.

2. Whisk together the milk, eggs, cheese, salt, dill, crushed red pepper flakes, paprika, and pepper in a large bowl. Using a spatula, mix in the cooked pasta.

3. Coat an oven-safe skillet with the olive oil, then pour the frittata batter into the skillet and spread it into an even layer.

4. Bake for 15 minutes, until golden brown. Remove from the oven, then chill for 10 minutes in the refrigerator before slicing and serving.

Caprese Chicken

Ingredients

- 2 tablespoons olive oil, divided

- 2 pounds boneless, skinless chicken breasts

- 1 teaspoon salt

- 1 teaspoon black pepper

- 1 teaspoon chili powder

- 1 tablespoon dried Italian seasoning

- 1 teaspoon sweet paprika

- 8 thick slices ripe tomato

- 8 (1-ounce) slices fresh mozzarella cheese

- 8 medium basil leaves

• 4 tablespoons balsamic glaze or balsamic reduction

Instructions

1. Preheat the oven to 350°F.

2. Heat a large cast-iron pan over medium heat and add 1 tablespoon of the olive oil.

3. While your oil is heating up, butterfly the chicken: cut each chicken breast from the side about three-quarters of the way through, then open the chicken and lay flat.

4. Rub each chicken breast with the remaining 1 tablespoon of olive oil and season with the salt, pepper, chili powder, Italian seasoning, and sweet paprika.

5. Place 2 slices of tomato, 2 slices of mozzarella cheese, and 2 basil leaves on one side of each

chicken breast. Close the chicken breasts and use toothpicks to help keep them closed around the filling.

6. Transfer the stuffed chicken breasts to the pan and sear for about 5 minutes on each side, until golden brown.

7. Transfer the pan to the oven until the internal temperature reaches 165°F.

8. Transfer the chicken breasts to a plate and let rest 3–5 minutes.

9. Slice into 1/4-inch slices and drizzle the balsamic glaze over the top of the chicken. Serve over your favorite salad.

Prosciutto Salad

Ingredients

- 7 ounces prosciutto, roughly chopped

- 2 cucumbers, diced

- 2 cups arugula, torn

- 1 cup halved cherry tomatoes

- 2 tablespoons extra-virgin olive oil

- 1 tablespoon mustard

- 1 tablespoon lemon juice

- 1/4 teaspoon dried oregano

- 1/4 teaspoon dried dill

- 1/4 teaspoon dried basil

Instructions

1. Combine the prosciutto, cucumbers, arugula, and cherry tomatoes in a medium bowl, tossing well.

2. Whisk the olive oil, mustard, lemon juice, oregano, dill, and basil together in a small bowl.

3. Pour the dressing over the prosciutto salad and toss to combine. Serve and enjoy!

DELIGHTFUL RECIPES FOR DINNER

Shephers Pie Boats

Ingredients

• 1 HMR Vegetable Stew with Beef Entree

• 1 Acorn squash

• 1 Cup peas

• 1 Cup mashed potatoes made with chicken broth

• Salt and pepper to taste

Instructions

1. Preheat oven to 350 degrees and prep baking sheet with aluminum foil and cooking spray.

2. Cut squash in half lengthwise and remove seeds. Then place flesh-side down and bake about 40 minutes (until tender).

3. While squash is baking, make mashed potatoes by boiling a couple of potatoes until tender.

4. Drain off water and add chicken broth to desired consistency, salt and pepper to taste, and mash together.

5. Combine entree with peas and warm in microwave for 1-2 minutes.

6. Put half the entree mixture in each of the squash halves, then top each half with a scoop of mashed potatoes.

7. Put back on baking sheet and bake another 10-15 minutes.

Super Spinach Lasagna

Ingredients

- 1 HMR Lasagna with Meat Sauce Entree

- 1 Cup frozen spinach, thawed and drained

- 1 Cup italian-style diced tomatoes

- 1 Cup fresh or canned mushrooms

Instructions

1. Cook and drain spinach according to package directions

2. Squeeze excess water from spinach

3. Layer spinach, tomatoes (reserving ¼ cup), mushrooms, and entree (if using fresh mushrooms, first saute in pan with non-stick cooking spray)

4. Microwave 2-3 minutes until heated

5. Top with remaining tomatoes

Whole Grain Medley in Squash

Ingredients

• 1 Acorn squash

• 1 HMR Whole Grain Medley with Chicken entree

Instructions

1. Preheat oven to 400 degrees and prep a baking sheet with parchment paper and spray with cooking spray.

2. Slice acorn squash in half and remove the seeds using a spoon.

3. Place the acorn squash flesh side down and bake for 40 minutes.

4. Heat entree as directed.

5. Once squash is cooked, evenly distribute the entree into both halves of the acorn squash.

Chicken and Broccoli Casserole

Ingredients

• 1 pound broccoli florets, steamed until just tender

• 2 cups seasoned shredded chicken

• 2 cups seasoned shredded chicken

• 1 cup cream cheese

• ¾ cup whipping cream

- ½ cup milk

- 1 tablespoon Dijon mustard

- 1 teaspoon minced garlic

- 1 cup shredded cheddar cheese

Instructions

1. Preheat oven to 375°F. Butter a 9-by-13-inch baking dish.

2. Combine the broccoli, chicken, and basil leaves in a bowl. Set aside.

3. Combine the cream cheese, cream, and milk in a saucepan over low heat, for about 5 minutes. Whisk in the mustard and garlic until smooth. Pour the cheese sauce over the chicken and broccoli mixture and toss to fully coat. Spread the mixture into the

prepared baking dish and cover with the shredded cheese.

4. Bake for 20–30 minutes, until hot throughout and the cheese has browned. Cool for 5 minutes then serve.

Chicken Parmesan Meatballs

Ingredients

• 14 ounces ground chicken

• ¾ cup shredded mozzarella cheese

• ⅔ cup shredded Parmesan cheese

• 1 zucchini, shredded

• 1 egg

• 2 teaspoons white onion, diced

• 2 teaspoons dried minced garlic

• 2 teaspoons dried basil

• 1 teaspoon salt

• 1 tablespoon ground pepper

• 1 cup marinara sauce

• ½ cup shredded cheddar cheese

Instructions

1. Preheat oven to 400°F. Grease a casserole dish with olive oil.

2. In a large bowl, combine all the Ingredients except for the marinara sauce and cheddar cheese, and mix thoroughly. Make about 24 meatballs and set apart.

3. In a skillet, add some olive oil and sear the meatballs. Place them in a casserole dish.

4. Bake in the oven for 20 minutes or until the meatballs are cooked through.

5. Remove from the oven and top with the sauce and cheese. Bake for another 10–15 minutes or until the cheese is melted. Serve hot.

Chicken Rolls

Ingredients

• 2 chicken breasts, flattened, grilled, and sliced

• ½ cup shredded mozzarella cheese

• 2 tablespoons minced chives

• 1 tablespoon lemon zest

• 2 tablespoons sesame seeds

• ½ avocado, thinly sliced

• ½ cucumber, sliced

• 2 tablespoons mayonnaise

Instructions

1. Place a piece of plastic wrap on the counter. Overlap the slices of chicken to form a rectangle.

2. Spread the mozzarella over the top of the chicken.

3. Place the sliced avocado and cucumbers in the center of the rectangle.

4. Top with minced chives, lemon zest, and sesame seeds.

5. Use the plastic wrap to help you roll the chicken. As if you are doing sushi rolls.

6. Once the rolls are ready, set them in the freezer for 30 minutes. Cut them into 12 pieces, 2 cm thick. Serve with mayonnaise.

Spanish Chicken and Rice

Ingredients

• ¼ cup dry white wine

• ¼ teaspoon saffron threads

• 2 teaspoons salt, divided

• 1 teaspoon black pepper, divided

• 4 bone-in, skin-on chicken thighs

• 1 tablespoon extra-virgin olive oil

- 1 medium onion, finely diced

- 1 red bell pepper, finely diced

- 1 medium carrot, diced

- 2 tablespoons minced garlic

- 1 bay leaf

- 2 cups chicken broth

- 1 cup short-grain rice

- ¾ cup frozen peas, thawed

- 2 tablespoons chopped parsley

Instructions

1. Preheat the oven to 375°F.

2. Combine the wine and saffron in a bowl and set aside.

3. Rub 1 teaspoon salt and ½ teaspoon pepper onto the chicken thighs, then set aside.

4. Heat the olive oil in a large oven-safe pan over medium-high heat.

5. Arrange the chicken thighs skin-side down in the pan and cook for 4 minutes, until browned. Turn the chicken over and cook for 4 more minutes, until golden brown on both sides, then transfer the chicken thighs to a plate.

6. Reduce the heat to medium-low and add the onion, bell pepper, carrot, and garlic to the pan. Cook, stirring frequently, for 5–7 minutes, until tender.

7. Stir in the wine–saffron mixture, the remaining 1 teaspoon salt and ½ teaspoon pepper, and the bay leaf.

8. Cook for 5–10 minutes, until most of the wine has evaporated, then add the chicken thighs, chicken broth, and short-grain rice and bring to a simmer.

9. Cover the pan and place it in the oven. Bake for 30 minutes, until chicken is tender and the meatpulls apart.

10. Remove the pan from the oven and stir in the peas. Allow to cool for 5 minutes.11. Divide the chicken and rice between four serving bowls and top with parsley before serving. Refrigerate leftovers in an airtight container for up to 3 days.

Supreme Pizza

Ingredients

• 1 frozen cauliflower pizza crust

• ½ cup sugar-free pizza sauce

• 1–1½ cups shredded mozzarella cheese

• 1 cup cooked and crumbled ground beef or Italian sausage

• 2 tablespoons thinly sliced sweet onion

• 2 tablespoons thinly sliced green pepper

• 2 tablespoons chopped fresh mushrooms

Instructions

1. Preheat the oven to 425°F.

2. Place the crust on a baking sheet and bake for 10 minutes, until firm and beginning to crisp.

3. Remove from the oven and spread the sauce around the pizza crust, leaving a small border uncovered. Evenly distribute the cheese over the

sauce. Sprinkle the meat and vegetables evenly over the top.

4. Bake for another 5–10 minutes, until the toppings are hot and the cheese is beginning to brown.

5. Slice the pizza into 8 pieces and serve immediately.

Chicken, Chickpea, and Pita Salad

Ingredients

- 2 teaspoons ground sumac

- 1 teaspoon ground cumin

- 1 teaspoon dried oregano

- 4 tablespoons extra-virgin olive oil, divided

- 2 tablespoons lemon juice, divided

- 1 lemon, sliced

- 4 boneless, skinless chicken breast fillets

- 1 (8-inch) whole-wheat pita, sliced

- 1 (15-ounce) can chickpeas, rinsed and drained

- 2 cups chopped parsley

- 1 red onion, thinly sliced

- ¼ cup crumbled feta cheese

Instructions

1. Combine the sumac, cumin, oregano, 1 tablespoon of the olive oil, 1 tablespoon of the lemon juice, and the lemon slices in a medium bowl.

2. Add the chicken and toss to combine. Cover with plastic wrap and refrigerate for 20 minutes.

3. When ready to cook the chicken, preheat the oven to 360°F.

4. Heat 1 tablespoon of the olive oil in a large oven-safe pan over medium-high heat.

5. Add the chicken breasts and cook for 2 minutes on each side, until both sides are lightly golden.

6. Transfer the pan to the oven and bake for 8 minutes, or until the chicken reaches an internal temperature of 165°F.

7. When the chicken is cooked through, remove the pan from the oven, loosely cover it with aluminum foil, and allow the chicken to rest for 2 minutes.

8. Heat 1 tablespoon of olive oil in another pan over medium-high heat.

9. Add the pita slices and cook for 2 minutes per side, until golden brown. Remove the pita bread from the pan and set aside.

10. Add the chickpeas to the same pan and stir for 2 minutes, until heated through. Set aside.

11. Slice the chicken and place it in a large bowl with the chickpeas, pita, parsley, onion, and feta. Toss to combine.

12. Drizzle the remaining 1 tablespoon olive oil and 1 tablespoon lemon juice over the top.

13. Divide the salad between four serving bowls and enjoy! Refrigerate leftovers in an airtight container for up to 3 days.

Turkey Burgers

Ingredients

- 1 pound ground turkey

- 1 large egg

- ½ cup finely ground almond flour

- ¼ cup sweet onion, minced

- ¼ cup fresh basil, chopped

- 1 tablespoon garlic, minced

- 1 tablespoon olive oil

- ¼ tbsp pink Himalayan salt

Instructions

1. Combine all the Ingredients in a bowl and gently mix to fully incorporate. Shape the meat mixture into 4 equal-sized patties.

2. To cook on the stovetop, heat the olive oil in a frying pan over medium-high heat. Add the burgers and cook for 4 minutes on each side, or until the turkey reaches an internal temperature of 160°F. To grill, heat the grill to medium-high. Coat the grill grates and burgers with olive oil to prevent the meat from sticking to the grates. Grill for 6–7 minutes on each side.

3. Serve immediately or refrigerate in an airtight container for up to 3 days.

Vegetarian Greek Pasta

Ingredients

- 1 cup cherry tomatoes

- 1 medium onion, diced

- 1 medium red bell pepper, diced

- 4 garlic cloves, minced

- ½ cup loosely packed fresh basil leaves

- ¼ cup loosely packed fresh oregano

- ¼ cup pitted and sliced kalamata olives

- 2 tablespoons extra-virgin olive oil, divided

- ½ tablespoon salt

- 1½ cups crumbled rennet-free feta cheese

- 1 teaspoon black pepper

- 1 pound dry rigatoni pasta

Instructions

1. Preheat the oven to 350°F.

2. Combine the tomatoes, onion, bell pepper, garlic, basil, oregano, and olives in a baking dish. Drizzle

with 1 tablespoon of the olive oil, sprinkle with the salt, and toss to combine.

3. Place the feta in the middle of the tomato mixture and drizzle the remaining tablespoon of olive oil on top of the cheese. Sprinkle with the black pepper.

4. Bake for 40 minutes, until the tomatoes burst. Remove from the oven and allow to cool for 5 minutes.

5. Meanwhile, cook the rigatoni pasta according to the manufacturer's Instructions, reserving 1 cup of the pasta water before draining.

6. Drain the pasta and transfer to a large bowl. Mash the feta and tomato mixture with a fork and mix until combined, then add the feta-tomato sauce to the bowl with the pasta. Mix until combined, adding in the reserved pasta water if necessary.

7. Divide the rigatoni between four serving plates and enjoy! Refrigerate leftovers in an airtight container for up to 5 days.

Zucchini Boats

Ingredients

• 1 teaspoon olive oil

• ½ cup chopped sweet onion

• 1 tablespoon minced garlic

• 1 pound ground turkey

• 2 medium zucchinis, sliced in half lengthwise

• 1 (28-ounce) can diced tomatoes

• ½ cup pitted and chopped kalamata olives

• 1 cup crumbled feta cheese

Instructions

1. Preheat the oven to 400°F

2. Heat the olive oil in a frying pan over medium heat. Add the onion and garlic and sauté 3 minutes, until soft. Add the ground turkey and cook, stirring, 10–13 minutes, until the turkey is cooked through.

3. Meanwhile, scoop out the insides of the zucchini halves, leaving a thin layer of flesh and skin intact. Chop the zucchini insides and add to the pan with the turkey mixture. Cook for 4 minutes, until the zucchini is tender. Add half the tomatoes and all the olives. Cook just until heated through.

4. Spread the remaining half of the tomatoes on the bottom of a 9-by-13-inch baking dish. Place the zucchini halves on top, skin side down. Divide the

turkey mixture between the 4 zucchini halves and top with the feta cheese.

5. Cover with foil and bake for 20 minutes, then uncover and bake for 15 minutes more, until the cheese is golden and filling is hot throughout. Serve immediately.

Mudardara and Side Salad

Ingredients

• 1 cup brown lentils

• 5 cups water, divided

• 1 cup rice

• 2 tablespoons extra-virgin olive oil

• 1 large onion, roughly chopped

- ½ tablespoon salt

- 1 large tomato, diced

- 1 large cucumber, diced

- 1 medium onion, diced

- 1 cup chopped parsley

- Juice of 1 lemon

- ½ cup water

- 1 teaspoon extra-virgin olive oil

- 1 tablespoon dried mint

- 1 teaspoon chili flakes

- ½ tablespoon salt

Instructions

1. Combine the lentils and 3 cups of the water in a pot over medium-high heat. Simmer covered for 20 minutes, until the lentils become tender. Stir occasionally, if needed.

2. Add the rice and the remaining 2 cups of water and cook over low heat covered for 15–25 minutes, until the liquid has evaporated and the rice is tender. Remove the pot from the heat and set aside.

3. Heat the olive oil in a skillet over medium-high heat and add the onions and salt. Stir for 5–8 minutes, until the onions have caramelized, then remove from the heat.

4. Stir the caramelized onions and their oil into the lentil-rice mixture and set aside.

5. To assemble the salad, combine the tomato, cucumber, onion, parsley, lemon juice, water, olive oil, mint, chili flakes, and salt in a bowl.

6. Place the mudardara in a serving dish and top with the salad. Serve immediately. Refrigerate leftovers in an airtight container for up to 5 days.

Moghrabieh with Chicken

Ingredients

• 1 (2–3 pound) whole chicken

• 3 teaspoons salt, divided

• 1 teaspoon black pepper, divided

• 1 teaspoon Lebanese seven-spice blend

• ¼ cup plus 2 tablespoons extra-virgin olive oil, divided

• 2 garlic cloves

• 1 (2-inch) cinnamon stick

• 2 bay leaves

• 1 teaspoon whole cloves

• 2 cups peeled pearl onions

• 1 teaspoon ground cinnamon

• 1 teaspoon ground cumin

• 1 (15-ounce) can chickpeas, drained and rinsed

• 2 cups dry moghrabieh

Instructions

1. Sprinkle the chicken with 1 teaspoon of the salt, ½ teaspoon of the pepper, and the seven-spice blend.

2. Heat 2 tablespoons of the olive oil in a large Dutch-oven pot over medium-high heat.

3. Add the chicken, breast side down, and cook for 4 minutes, until golden brown.

4. Turn the chicken over and cook for 4 minutes more, until golden on both sides.

5. Add enough water to cover the chicken, then add the garlic, cinnamon stick, bay leaves, and cloves.

6. Cook the chicken uncovered for 30 minutes, removing any fat that rises to the surface with a spoon.

7. After 30 minutes, add the pearl onions, stir to combine, and cook the chicken for another 15 minutes.

8. Whisk the cinnamon, cumin, and remaining ½ teaspoon pepper together in a bowl. Set aside one-quarter of the cinnamon mixture.

9. Add the remaining three-quarters of the spice mixture and the chickpeas to the chicken. Cook for another 10 minutes, then add the remaining 2 teaspoons salt.

10. Fill another pot with water and bring to a boil over medium-high heat. Add the dry moghrabieh and cook for 15–20 minutes, until tender.

11. Place the moghrabieh over medium-low heat and cook, stirring, for 3–4 minutes, until fluffed up.

12. Drain the moghrabieh, then return it to the pot and add the remaining ¼ cup olive oil and the reserved seasoning mixture.

13. Add a few ladles of the chicken broth to the moghrabieh and continue to cook for 7–10 minutes more, allowing the pearl couscous to absorb the chicken flavor.

14. Divide the moghrabieh between six serving bowls, adding a few ladles of the chicken broth. Add some of the chicken, onions, and chickpeas to the moghrabieh in each bowl. Serve and enjoy! Refrigerate leftovers in an airtight container for up to 3 days.

Mediterranean Turkey Casserole

Ingredients

• ½ pound ground turkey

• ½ cup chopped green bell pepper

• 1 shallot, chopped

• 1 cup rinsed, drained, and chopped canned artichoke hearts

• 1 cup chopped broccoli florets

• 1 medium zucchini, sliced

• 6 large eggs

• 6 large egg whites

• 3 tablespoons fat-free milk

• 1 teaspoon Italian seasoning

• ¼ teaspoon garlic powder

• ¼ teaspoon black pepper

• ⅓ cup crumbled feta cheese

Instructions

1. Preheat the oven to 350°F and coat a 9-inch square baking dish with nonstick cooking spray.

2. Combine the ground turkey, green pepper, and shallots in a skillet over medium heat. Cook for 8–10 minutes, stirring occasionally, until there are no pink streaks remaining in the turkey.

3. Drain the turkey–veggie mixture and transfer to the prepared baking dish.

4. Arrange the artichokes, broccoli, and zucchini slices on top of the turkey.

5. Whisk the eggs, egg whites, milk, Italian seasoning, garlic powder, and pepper together in a large bowl until well combined.

6. Pour the egg mixture over the turkey–veggie mixture, then sprinkle the feta cheese on top.

7. Bake, uncovered, for 45–50 minutes, until golden.

8. Remove from the oven and allow to cool for 10 minutes.

9. Divide the casserole between six serving dishes and enjoy! Refrigerate leftovers in an airtight container for up to 3 days.

DELIGHTFUL RECIPES FOR SNACKS

Fiesta Chicken Burrito Bowl

Ingredients

• 1 HMR Fiesta Chicken Entree

• 2 cups mixed green lettuce

• 1/4 cup corn

• 1/4 cup black beans

• 1/4 cup diced red bell pepper

• 1/4 cup diced green bell pepper

• 2 Tbsp. diced red onion

• 1/2 cup sliced radishes

- 1/2 cup sliced cucumber

- Optional: cilantro for topping

Instructions

1. Heat entrée according to package.

2. Mix entree with vegetables (vegetables can be warm or cold) and top with cilantro.

Fajita Bowl

Ingredients

- 1/2 cup sliced onions

- 1/2 cup sliced bell pepper

- 1 HMR Chicken with Barbecue Sauce Entree

- 1/4 packet fajita seasoning

• 1/4 cup water

• Juice from 1/2 lime

• 1/4 cup salsa (optional)

Instructions

1. Place a pan over medium heat and spray with cooking spray. Add onions and peppers. Slice chicken into strips and add to pan. Heat until soft, about 5-10 minutes.

2. Dissolve seasoning in water and add to pan with lime juice, if desired. Mix together and heat until warm.

3. Add rice and beans from entree and stir thoroughly. Remove from heat and top with salsa.

Chocolate Chunkie Monkie Shake

Ingredients

- 1 HMR Chocolate Shake

- 1 tbsp. PB2 Peanut Butter Flavor

- 1 whole ripe banana

- 1 cup water

- 6 ice cubes

Instructions

1. Pour 8 oz cold water into blender; turn blender on low speed.

2. Add HMR chocolate shake, PB2 and banana; turn blender up to medium speed.

3. Add six ice cubes, one at a time. Turn blender up to high speed and continue to blend for 2 minutes.

4. Pour into large cup and enjoy!

Cranberry Orange Shake

Ingredients

- 1 HMR vanilla shake

- 1 Cup fresh cranberries

- 1 12oz can diet orange soda

- 5 ice cubes

Instructions

1. Add all Ingredients to a blender and blend until smooth.

Green Giant Shake

Ingredients

- 1 HMR vanilla shake

- 1 Cup water

- 1 Cup fresh spinach

- 1/4 Avocado

- 1/2 pear or 1/2 cup pineapple (sliced)

- 4-6 ice cubes

Instructions

1. Add Ingredients to blender and blend until smooth.

Mint Hot Chocolate

Ingredients

• 2 Cups hot water

• 1 HMR Chocolate Shake

• 1 Tbs sugar-free chocolate pudding mix

• 1 Drop peppermint extract

Instructions

1. Heat 2 cups of water until warm (not boiling).

2. Add hot water to blender with chocolate shake, sugar-free chocolate pudding mix, and peppermint extract.

3. Blend until smooth.

Pumpkin Pie Smoothie

Ingredients

- 1 HMR vanilla shake

- 1 cup water

- 1/2-1 banana

- 1/4 cup canned pumpkin

- 1 tsp cinnamon

- 1/4 tsp ginger (optional)

- 1/4 tsp nutmeg (optional)

- 1/2 tsp vanilla extract

- Dash of salt

- 4 ice cubes

Instructions

1. Add all Ingredients to blender and blend until smooth.

Chili Fries

Ingredients

- 1 HMR Turkey Chili with Beans Entree

- 1 large white (russett) or sweet potato, cut to fries

- 1 Tbsp. cheese flavoring (powdered)

- 1/8 tsp. salt / seasoning (to taste)

- 1 tsp. hot sauce (optional)

Instructions

1. Place a pan over medium-high heat and add potato slices (fries) and salt, cook until lightly browned.

2. Put 'fried' potatoes on microwave safe plate and top with Turkey Chili entree and cheese flavoring.

3. Microwave for 1 minute.

4. For additional kick, add hot sauce.

Caramel Apple Shake

Ingredients

• 1 HMR vanilla shake

• 1 Cup water

• 1 Apple (chopped)

• 2 tsp sugar-free caramel syrup

- 1 tsp cinnamon

- 4 ice cubes

Instructions

1. Peel and chop apple.

2. Add all Ingredients to a blender and blend until smooth

Berry Berry Good Shake

Ingredients

- 1 HMR Vanilla Shake

- 1/2 cup blueberries (fresh or frozen)

- 1/2 cup blackberries (fresh or frozen)

- 1 Tbs sugar-free white chocolate syrup

• 4-6 ice cubes (omit if using frozen fruit)

Instructions

1. Add Ingredients to blender and mix until smooth

Berry Banana Parfait

Ingredients

• 1 HMR Vanilla Shake

• 1 cup water

• 4-6 ice cubes

• 1 cup blueberries

• 1/2 cup blackberries or raspberries

• 1 banana, sliced

• 1 tsp chia seeds (optional for Phase 2)

Instructions

1. Add the vanilla shake, water, and ice to a blender and mix until smooth. Make it extra thick by adding more ice (6-8 cubes), and blending longer. Option to mix in 1 tsp. chia seeds for Phase 2.

2. Spoon 1/3 of your blended vanilla shake into the bottom of the glass (keeping the remaining 2/3 of the shake in the blender).

3. Add a layer of blueberries to the top of the shake in the glass (about 1/2 cup).

4. Add 1/2 cup blackberries or raspberries to the remaining shake in your blender and mix until smooth.

5. Spoon 1/3 of the blended shake on top of the layer of blueberries in your glass, then top with a layer of sliced bananas.

6. Add blueberries (about 1/3 cup) to the remaining shake left in the blender and mix until smooth.

7. Spoon the rest of the shake into your glass and top it off with remaining blueberries or raspberries and enjoy with a spoon!

Salted Caramel Mocha Shake

Ingredients

• 1 HMR Chocolate Shake

• 8 oz. water

• 1 tsp. sugar-free salted caramel syrup

• 1 tsp. vanilla extract

• 1 tsp. instant coffee mix

• 1 tsp. unsweetened cocoa powder

- 4 Ice cubes

- 1 packet Splenda (optional)

Instructions

1. Add Ingredients to blender and mix until smooth.

Strawberry Swirl Shake

Ingredients

- 1 HMR 120 Vanilla Shake (or HMR 70 Plus lactose-free Shake)

- 1 banana

- 1 cup strawberries (fresh or frozen)

- 6-8 oz water

- 4 ice cubes (omit if using frozen fruit)

Instructions

1. Add Ingredients to blender and mix until smooth.

Twice Baked Pot Pie Potatoes

Ingredients

• 1 HMR Crustless Chicken Pot Pie Entree

• 1 medium sweet potato

• 1 Tbsp. fat-free sour cream

• Optional: chives for topping

Instructions

1. Cook sweet potato (bake or microwave) and then slice down the middle.

2. Heat entree in microwave for about 1 minute, then pour over cooked sweet potato.

3. Top with fat-free sour cream and chives.

Vanilla Berry Smoothie Bowl

Ingredients

- 1 HMR vanilla shake or protein powder

- 1/2 Cup frozen cauliflower

- 1/2 Banana

- 1/2 tsp vanilla extract

- Dash of cinnamon

- 1/4 cup water

• Toppings: sliced banana, berries, almond butter, chia seeds

Instructions

1. Combine Ingredients in a blender and blend until smooth.

2. If mixture is too thick, add extra water 2 Tbs at a time.

3. Add blended smoothie to a bowl. It should be thick enough to eat with a spoon.

4. Top with desired toppings and enjoy!

5

SUCCESS STORIES, TIPS AND REVIEWS

Success Stories and Tips from Real People

Susan, a teacher and mom from Boston who started using HMR in April 2019, is a satisfied customer.

"My experience with HMR has been great," she says. "I quickly and easily lost over 50 pounds and have been maintaining that weight loss for over 2.5 years."

Here's what Susan finds most helpful:

The support. "Weekly coaching is included in the price, the Facebook group is, obviously, free and my coach is available for extra coaching via email or phone whenever I need it."

The convenience. "The food is shipped to my front door, and it's so easy to prepare and pack for a day away from home."

Never have to feel deprived. "On HMR you can eat as much as you want, as long as what you are eating is a healthy choice."

Although it was challenging for her to adjust to eating differently than her family, she's pleased with her successful experience with HMR.

"I am very happy with my results," she says.

Susan shares her success tips:

Focus on what you can do instead of what you can't. This attitude shift allowed Susan to stay in phase 2 of the program for far longer than any other program she's been on.

Keep yourself accountable. Tracking your activities and progress on the HMR app every day and attending each weekly Zoom call will keep you connected to your health behaviors and goals.

Practice healthy, sustainable habits for life-long success. Utilize phase 2 long term to help you keep the weight off forever.

Eating Out

You'll want to avoid eating out altogether in phase 1. Even if restaurants allow you to bring your own HMR foods and prepare them, you're advised to control your environment and stay out of temptation's way.

Tips for staying on track in "challenging" food environments, like parties, include:

- Eating before you go.
- Bringing your own food.
- Keeping a list of restaurants with enjoyable low-calorie options for Phase 2.

Reviews

Despite faring better in past years, the HMR program did not even make the list for the U.S. News & World Report's Best Diets 2023 rankings. WW (formerly Weight Watchers), the Jenny Craig diet, and Noom took the top three spots for best commercial diets. U.S. News & World Report dinged HMR for the potential monotony of the diet without customization and limited allowance for eating out.

There is limited scientific evidence that backs up the weight loss results of the HMR program. One small study found that participants with obesity who took part in an HMR-style diet (eating meal replacements and fruits and vegetables) lost an average of 37.4 pounds over 18 weeks.

Another small study found that a low-cal plan with three shakes, two meal replacements, and five servings of fruits and veggies daily helped dieters with obesity lose an average of 28.6 pounds more than control group participants, who received weight management counseling only.

U.S. News Expert Reviews:

"Safety of this diet is uncertain and can result in renal issues, especially in patients with impaired kidney function."

William Yancy, MD

"The HMR diet offers a structured and easily followed plan, which can be of great assistance to individuals who encounter difficulties when making food choices independently. HMR meal replacements are convenient and entail minimal preparation, which may prove attractive to individuals leading hectic lives or those who encounter challenges in preparing healthy meals."

Steph Grasso, MS, RD

"HMR is fine for the short term and will lead to weight loss, but no shake or packaged meal can replace a variety of wholesome foods."

Jill Weisenberger, MS, RDN, CDCES, CHWC, FAND

"The HMR program's inclusion of health coaching, online support and physical activity is commendable, but its reliance on meal replacements and prepackaged products knocks it down several notches."

Michael Greger, PhD, RDN, CDN

www.ingramcontent.com/pod-product-compliance
Lightning Source LLC
Chambersburg PA
CBHW061041250726

48653CB00001B/200